INFUSING WITH CANNABIS FOR NATURAL PAIN RELIEF

BY: MMJ_DAVID (DAVID YRIGOYEN LLC)

TABLE OF CONTENTS

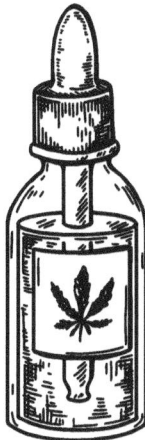

I0105674

MMJ_DAVID

INTRODUCTION: THE HISTORY OF CANNABIS USE

🌿 THE HISTORY OF CANNABIS USED AS A MEDICINE HAS BEEN LINKED AS FAR BACK AS 2900 BC.

🌿 "THE CHINESE EMPEROR FU HIS (CA. 2900 BC), WHOM THE CHINESE CREDIT WITH BRINGING CIVILIZATION TO CHINA, SEEMS TO HAVE MADE REFERENCE TO MA, THE CHINESE WORD FOR CANNABIS, NOTING THAT CANNABIS WAS VERY POPULAR MEDICINE THAT POSSESSED BOTH YIN AND YANG."- ROBERT DEITCH HEMP: AMERICAN HISTORY REVISITED: THE PLANT WITH A DIVIDED HISTORY, 2003

🌿 THE FIRST REPORTS OF CANNABIS BEING INGESTED DATE BACK TO INDIA 1000 BC, IN THE FORM OF BHANG.

🌿 "BHANG, A CANNABIS DRINK GENERALLY MIXED WITH MILK, IS USED AS AN ANESTHETIC AND ANTI-PHLEGMATIC IN INDIA. CANNABIS BEGINS TO BE USED IN INDIA TO TREAT A WIDE VARIETY OF HUMAN MALADIES,"- US NATIONAL COMMISSION ON MARIHUANA AND DRUG ABUSE MARIHUANA, A SIGNAL OF MISUNDERSTANDING

🌿 IN 1850 MARIJUANA WAS ADDED TO US PHARMACOPEIA

🌿 1942 MARIJUANA REMOVED FROM US PHARMACOPEIA

OPENING INTRODUCTION

THIS BOOK WAS CREATED WITH LOVE AND INTENT.

CANNABIS HAS BEEN A PART OF MY LIFE FOR OVER 30 YEARS. SINCE 2011 I HAVE BEEN HELPING PEOPLE FIND NATURAL RELIEF WITH CANNABIS.

CANNABIS CAN BE USED IN DIFFERENT WAYS THAT HAVE DIFFERENT BENEFITS. THIS BOOK WILL GIVE YOU AN INTRODUCTION TO CANNABIS AS A MEDICINE, AND WILL GIVE YOU KNOWLEDGE ON HOW TO USE AND MAKE CANNABIS INFUSED PRODUCTS AT HOME WITH EASE AND CONFIDENCE.

WHEN MAKING THIS BOOK, I WAS AT A POINT IN MY LIFE WHERE I WAS IN CHRONIC PAIN AND NEEDED RELIEF THROUGHOUT THE DAY. CANNABIS WAS MY MEDICINE OF CHOICE FOR PAIN RELIEF, BUT I COULDN'T BE IN A STATE THAT WOULDN'T ALLOW ME TO WORK AT A HIGH LEVEL. THAT IS WHEN I LEARNED ABOUT THC-A AND HOW BENEFICIAL IT IS FOR INFLAMMATION, ALONG WITH OTHER CANNABINOIDS LIKE CBD AND CBN.

THERE IS A LOT MORE I WOULD LOVE TO ADD TO THIS BOOK, BUT I WANTED TO MAKE IT READER FRIENDLY AND EASY TO FOLLOW. I WILL PUT OUT MORE PUBLICATIONS ON THE EXPERIENCES I, AND OTHERS, HAVE HAD WITH CANNABIS. FOR NOW, ENJOY THIS BOOK AND I PRAY YOU LEARN SOMETHING THAT CAN HELP YOU OR OTHERS ALONG THIS JOURNEY.

INITIAL PUBLICATION IN 2015

MMJ_DAVID

DISCLAIMER

THIS BOOK IS NOT INTENDED FOR MEDICAL PURPOSES. THIS BOOK IS SHARED INFORMATION THAT HAS BEEN AROUND FOR THOUSANDS OF YEARS, AND HAS BEEN KNOWN IN THE UNITED STATES FOR HUNDREDS OF YEARS. NOW, WITH SCIENCE AND RESEARCH, WE ARE ABLE TO CONFIRM THE MEDICINAL BENEFITS OF CANNABIS.

I AM NOT A DOCTOR, I AM NOT A HEALTHCARE PROFESSIONAL. I AM A CANNABIS ADVOCATE, A NATURAL MEDICINE ADVOCATE, AND A HEALTH ENTHUSIAST.

THROUGH MY JOURNEY I HAVE BEEN ABLE TO FIND RELIEF WITH CANNABIS, NATURE, AND ALTERNATIVE THERAPIES LIKE ACUPUNTURE, MASSAGE THERAPY AND MORE.

CANNABIS IS NOT A CURE ALL, AT THE MOMENT, BUT IT DOES HELP MORE THAN SOME OF THESE CHEMICAL POISONS THAT ARE ALLOWED TO BE SOLD OPENLY AND FREELY.

FREE THE PLANT AND HEALTH IS WEALTH!

IF YOU ARE LOOKING TO USE CANNABIS AS AN ALTERNATIVE, CONSULT A HEALTHCARE PROFESSIONAL LIKE THE NATUROPATHIC DOCTORS AT NATURAL HEALING CARE CENTER

NATURALHEALINGCARECENTER.COM

MMJ_DAVID

INTRODUCTION: THE HISTORY OF CANNABIS USE CONT'D

🌿 CANNABIS CAN BE USED IN DIFFERENT WAYS LIKE: INHALATION (SMOKING OR VAPORIZING), INGESTING (EDIBLES, TINCTURES, CAPSULES), TOPICALS (RUBS, OILS, SALVES, BALMS), SUPPOSITORIES, AND MORE.

🌿 THE EARLIEST FORMS OF USING CANNABIS WERE BY INGESTION AND TOPICAL APPLICATION WITH BODY OILS, THIS WAS BECAUSE OF THE CONVENIENCE FACTOR. SMOKING CANNABIS WAS NOT AS EASY THOUSANDS OF YEARS AGO.

🌿 THERE ARE WAYS TO USE CANNABIS WITHOUT ANY PSYCHOACTIVE EFFECTS WITH EDIBLES AND TOPICALS, OR EVEN CERTAIN CANNABINOIDS. WE WILL TALK ABOUT THAT MORE IN THIS BOOK.

🌿 EVERY PERSON, AND MAMMAL, HAS AN ENDOCANNABINOID SYSTEM THAT BINDS TO THE CANNABINOIDS IN CANNABIS. WE ARE GENETICALLY MADE TO USE THIS PLANT.

🌿 HOW YOU INTAKE THE CANNABIS WILL DEPEND ON THE RELIEF YOU WILL OBTAIN.

🌿 NOT ONE PERSON HAS EVER DIED FROM OVER CONSUMING CANNABIS. IF YOU DO OVER CONSUME CANNABIS: RELAX, DRINK PLENTY OF WATER, TRY TO EAT SOMETHING, YOU MIGHT EVEN HAVE TO REGURGITATE, BUT IT WILL WEAR OFF.

INTRODUCTION: CANNABINOIDS AND THE ENDOCANNABINOID SYSTEM

🍁 CANNABIS CONTAINS CANNABINOIDS. THE MOST COMMON ARE THC (DELTA-9-TETRAHYDROCANNABINOL), CBD (CANNABIDIOL), CBN (CANNABINOL), AND CBC (CANNABICHROMENE).

🍁 CANNABINOIDS ARE A CLASS OF DIVERSE CHEMICAL COMPOUNDS THAT ACT ON RECEPTORS IN THE ENDOCANNABINOID SYSTEM.

🍁 THE ENDOCANNABINOID SYSTEM IS MADE UP OF DIFFERENT RECEPTORS (CB1, CB2, CBX, GPR55, MORE?) THAT NATURALLY BOND TO THE CANNABINOIDS IN CANNABIS. CB1 RECEPTORS ACT ON OUR NERVOUS SYSTEM, CB2 RECEPTORS ACT ON OUR IMMUNE SYSTEM AND ARE ALSO IN OUR SKIN. THE ENDOCANNABINOID SYSTEM WAS DISCOVERED BY DR. MECHOULAM IN HIS LAB IN INDIA IN 1992, BECAUSE OF PROHIBITION US RESEARCH ON CANNABIS AND THE ENDOCANNABINOID SYSTEM IN MINIMAL AND DONE IN INDEPENDENT LABS

INTRODUCTION: CANNABINOIDS AND THE ENDOCANNABINOID SYSTEM (CONT'D)

🍁 CANNABIS ALSO CONTAINS TERPENES, TERPENES ARE A LARGE CLASS OF ORGANIC HYDROCARBONS PRODUCED BY A WIDE VARIETY OF PLANTS, THEY ARE ALSO REFERRED TO AS TERPENOIDS WHEN DENATURED BY OXIDATION (DRY AND CURE). THEY ARE THE MAIN BUILDING BLOCK OF ANY PLANT RESIN OR "ESSENTIAL OILS" AND CONTRIBUTE TO THE SCENT, FLAVOR AND COLORS. SOME ARE KNOWN TO HAVE MEDICINAL VALUE.- MMJDAVID.COM

🍁 WHEN USING CANNABIS AS MEDICINE, IT IS BEST TO INTAKE ALL THE CANNABINOIDS DAILY, THIS IS KNOWN AS THE ENTOURAGE EFFECT. WHEN THE CANNABINOIDS ARE ISOLATED THEY ARE NOT AS EFFECTIVE AS WHEN USED TOGETHER, SOME CANNABINOIDS COUNTER ACT THE ADVERSE EFFECTS OF OTHERS (EX. CBD REDUCES THE PSYCHOACTIVE EFFECTS AND ANXIETY CAUSED BY OVER CONSUMPTION OF THC).

🍁 THC IS THE CANNABINOID RESPONSIBLE FOR THE PSYCHOACTIVE (EUPHORIA) EFFECT OF CANNABIS, IT ALSO REDUCES PAIN RELIEF, NAUSEA, MUSCLE SPASMS, SEIZURES, PROMOTES NEW BRAIN CELL GROWTH, AND HELPS CANCER CELLS GO INTO APOPTOSIS. IT IS ALSO A GREAT MOOD ELEVATOR AND AUDITORY ENHANCER.

INTRODUCTION: CANNABINOIDS AND THE ENDOCANNABINOID SYSTEM (CONT'D)

🍁 THC-A IS NON-PSYCHOACTIVE AND IS VERY BENEFICIAL FOR REDUCING INFLAMMATION, PAIN RELIEF, SEIZURES AND CONVULSIONS, AND INHIBITING TUMOR AND CANCER CELL GROWTH.

🍁 CBD IS ALSO NON-PSYCHOACTIVE AND IS GREAT FOR PAIN RELIEF AND MUSCLE SPASMS, IT CAN ALSO BE USED TO TREAT SEIZURES, PARKINSON'S DISEASE AND CERTAIN CANCERS . CBD COUNTER ACTS THE ADVERSE EFFECTS OF THC (PARANOIA/ANXIETY WITH OVER CONSUMPTION) AND CAN HELP LENGTHEN THE PAIN RELIEF FROM THC. THERE ARE MANY MORE BENEFITS OF CBD HOWEVER, OVER CONSUMPTION CAN BE SEDATING.

🍁 CBD-A REDUCES INFLAMMATION AND INHIBITS TUMOR AND CANCER CELL GROWTH

🍁 CBN TREATS PAIN RELIEF AND MUSCLE SPASMS, IT ALSO ACTS AS A SLEEP AIDE.

YOU CAN LEARN MORE ABOUT THE INDIVIDUAL CANNABINOIDS ON MY PODCAST: TUESDAY NIGHT SMOKE SESH WITH MMJ_DAVID WE GO INTO FURTHER DEPTH ON CANNABINOIDS AND CANNABIS.

TOP 5 SECRETS TO BECOMING THE BEST CANNABIS CHEF YOU KNOW!

1) DOSING

2) DECARBOXYLATION

3) OIL VS BUTTER

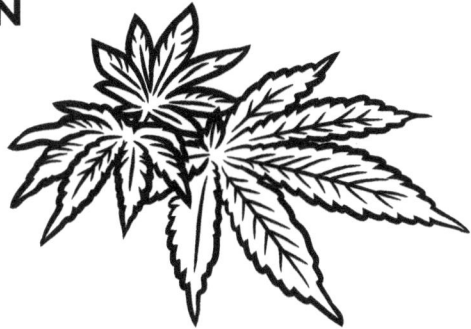

4)HEAT CONTROL

5) A.B.V

#1-DOSING

🌿 WHEN FIRST INGESTING CANNABIS IT IS BEST TO START SLOW, YOU CAN ALWAYS EAT MORE, BUT YOU CAN'T EAT LESS.

🌿 THE RECOMMENDED STARTING DOSE IS 2MG-5MG OF THC. THIS IS BECAUSE OF THE PSYCHOACTIVE EFFECTS OF THC, ALL OF THE OTHER CANNABINOIDS CAN BE CONSUMED AS MUCH AS NEEDED WITH LITTLE TO NO ADVERSE EFFECTS. OVER TIME YOU WILL START TO BUILD A TOLERANCE TOWARDS CANNABIS SO YOU MAY REQUIRE MORE CANNABINOIDS, EVERYBODY IS DIFFERENT AND REQUIRES DIFFERENT AMOUNTS BUT THIS IS A GOOD STARTING POINT.

🌿 THERE ARE TESTING CENTERS IN SOME STATES THAT WILL TEST YOUR PRODUCTS AND LET YOU KNOW THE SPECIFIC CANNABINOID BREAKDOWN. WITH THIS KNOWLEDGE YOU CAN TEST ALL YOUR HOMEMADE PRODUCTS FOR ACCURATE AT HOME DOSING.

#1-DOSING CONT'D
LET US DO A LITTLE MATH

🌿 EXAMPLE: IF THERE IS 20% THC IN A GRAM OF CANNABIS AND YOU USE 3.5 GRAMS (1/8TH OF CANNABIS) TO MAKE 8 OUNCES OF INFUSED OIL, THERE WILL BE CLOSE TO 700 MG OF THCA IN THE 8 OZ OF OIL, WHICH WILL BE CLOSE TO 2.9 MG THC IN 1 ML OF OIL.

🌿 20% THCA = 200MG THC PER GRAM

🌿 THAT WOULD EQUATE TO AROUND 700 MG OF THC IN 1/8TH OF CANNABIS FLOWER (OR 700 MG IN 1 CUP, BECAUSE WE ARE INFUSING 3.5 G IN 1 CUP OF OIL) WHICH WILL EQUAL TO ABOUT 2.9 MG THC IN 1 ML OF OIL.

🌿 1/8 OF CANNABIS IS 3.5 GRAMS

🌿 THERE ARE 8 OZ IN 1 CUP OF OIL OR BUTTER

🌿 THERE ARE 30 ML IN 1 OZ

🌿 20% THC = 200 MG OF THC PER GRAM OF CANNABIS FLOWER

200 MG * 3.5 G = 700 MG OF THC

700 MG / 8 OZ=87.5 MG OF THC PER 1 OZ OF OIL

87.5 MG / 30 ML= 2.9 MG OF THC PER 1 ML OF OIL OR BUTTER.

1 ML OF OIL OR BUTTER = 2.9 MG THC

#2-DECARBOXYLATION

🍁 DECARBOXYLATION IS THE REMOVAL OF A CARBON ATOM FROM THE CANNABINOIDS, FOR EXAMPLE DECARBOXYLATION OF THC-A (NON-PSYCHOACTIVE) CONVERTS IT TO THC (PSYCHOACTIVE).

🍁 THIS IS DONE WITH HEAT, THE CONVERSION HEAT NEEDED FOR THIS PROCESS IS 220 DEGREES FAHRENHEIT. WHEN SMOKED, THE FLAME AND HEAT FROM THE LIGHTER CONVERT THE THC-A TO THC AND THAT IS WHAT IS RESPONSIBLE FOR THE "HIGH" FEELING ASSOCIATED WITH CANNABIS USE. WHEN COOKING YOU NEED TO MANUALLY DECARBOXYLATE THE CANNABIS IF YOU WANT ANY PSYCHOACTIVE EFFECT. (***THIS PROCESS IF OPTIONAL***)

🍁 DECARBOXYLATION PROCESS:

🍁 USE A CANNABIS GRINDER (NOT COFFEE GRINDER) TO GROUND UP YOUR CANNABIS BUD MATERIAL.

🍁 SPREAD EVENLY ON COOKING TRAY OR FLAT HEAT SAFE TRAY

🍁 PRE-HEAT OVEN TO 225°F, ONCE HEATED PLACE TRAY OF CANNABIS INSIDE OVEN FOR 30 MINUTES.

🍁 REMOVE AND LET COOL FOR 5-10 MINUTES

#2-DECARBOXYLATION CONT'D

NOW YOUR CANNABIS HAS GONE THROUGH THE DECARBOXYLATION PROCESS AND YOU HAVE CONVERTED YOUR THC-A TO DELTA-9-THC (THE PSYCHOACTIVE CANNABINOID OF CANNABIS) AND IS READY TO INFUSE, INGEST, OR EVEN INHALE.

THE DECARBOXYLATION PROCESS WILL ALSO OCCUR IF YOU INFUSE YOUR OIL, OR BUTTER WITH THE 'RAW' CANNABIS FLOWER AND ADD HEAT OVER 225°F TO IT LATER (EX. BAKING COOKIES OR BROWNIES). THIS WILL CONVERT YOUR THC-A OIL TO DELTA-9-THC

AS MENTIONED EARLIER, IT IS BEST TO START LOW WHEN DOSING CANNABIS, ESPECIALLY WHEN INGESTING DELTA-9-THC. 10MG - 20MG AND MORE OF DELTA-9-THC CAN BE UNCOMFORTABLE FOR MOST PEOPLE. IF YOU DO INGEST TOO MUCH DELTA-9-THC, JUST RELAX AND TRY TO REST AND DRINK PLENTY OF WATER. THE EFFECTS WILL START TO LOWER AFTER A LITTLE BIT OF TIME AND YOU SHOULD FEEL BETTER IN A FEW HOURS.

DELTA-9-THC CAN PRODUCE A BIT OF A 'HANGOVER' EFFECT IF YOU OVER INGEST, BUT THAT WILL CLEAR UP BY THE END OF THE DAY.

NOBODY HAS EVER DIED FROM OVER CONSUMING CANNABIS OR DELTA-9-THC.

#3-OIL VS BUTTER

🌿 THE CANNABINOIDS IN CANNABIS BOND TO FATTY LIPID CELLS, THEREFORE A HIGHER FAT CONTENT ADDS MORE POTENCY. BUTTER IS REALLY HIGH IN FATS AND EASILY ABSORBS THE CANNABINOIDS, HOWEVER THERE ARE ALSO HEALTH PROBLEMS ASSOCIATED WITH THE OVER CONSUMPTION OF BUTTER AND THERE ARE PATIENTS WITH DIET RESTRICTIONS AND ALLERGIES TOWARDS BUTTER.

🌿 COCONUT OIL IS ALSO VERY HIGH IN FATS AND ABSORBS THE CANNABINOIDS WELL, COCONUT OIL ALSO HAS A LONGER SHELF LIFE THEN BUTTER AND CAN BE STORED IN A COOL DARK PLACE, UNLIKE BUTTER WHICH HAS A SHELF LIFE AND HAS TO BE STORED IN THE FRIDGE. COCONUT OIL IS ALSO GREAT FOR HEART DISEASE, BRAIN DISEASE, STRESS RELIEF, CANCER, THE IMMUNE SYSTEM, DIGESTION, WEIGHT LOSS, SKIN AND HAIR CARE AND MUCH MORE. COCONUT OIL IS RECOMMENDED TO BE CONSUMED DAILY.

🌿 THERE ARE OTHER OILS, FATS, AND DAIRY FREE BUTTERS THAT CAN BE USED, SOMETIMES IT COMES DOWN TO PERSONAL PREFERENCE.

#4-HEAT CONTROL

✻ WHEN COOKING YOUR OIL OR BUTTER IT IS IMPORTANT TO SIMMER AT A LOW TO MEDIUM HEAT, IF YOU EXCEED 225°F YOU RISK BURNING YOUR PRODUCT. THIS IS ALSO IMPORTANT TO KNOW FOR WHEN YOU ARE BAKING AND COOKING WITH YOUR COMPLETED PRODUCT, IF YOU SMELL BURNING OIL OR HEAVY VAPORIZED CANNABIS YOU WANT TO LOWER YOUR HEAT IMMEDIATELY (IF THE OIL/BUTTER IS BOILING, REMOVE FROM HEAT UNTIL IT COOLS AND LOWER TEMPERATURE). ***IT IS BEST TO KEEP A COOKING THERMOMETER NEARBY***

✻ THIS BOOK RECOMMENDS COOKING YOUR OIL AT 160°F-180°F, THIS WILL ALLOW YOU TO KEEP YOUR MATERIAL IN THE ACIDIC FORM (THC-A). IF YOU WANT TO ACTIVATE YOUR FINISHED PRODUCT YOU CAN DO SO BY BAKING IT IN YOUR FOOD (EX. COOKIES AND BROWNIES), THE HEAT FROM THE OVEN WILL ACTIVATE YOUR MATERIAL, HOWEVER YOU STILL DON'T WANT TO COOK THE MATERIAL AT HIGH HEATS. *AS MENTIONED ON PAGE 9*

#5-A.B.V

A.B.V (ALREADY BEEN VAPORIZED) IS MATERIAL THAT HAS ALREADY BEEN VAPORIZED. THE CANNABIS CAN BE PRICEY AND PATIENTS IN CHRONIC PAIN OR WITH OTHER CHRONIC CONDITIONS CAN REQUIRE A LOT OF CANNABIS USE, UNFORTUNATELY THE MARKET IS WHERE IT IS BUT THERE ARE WAYS TO SAVE. ONE WAY TO SAVE MONEY IS BY FIRST VAPORIZING YOUR PLANT MATERIAL WITH A VAPORIZER (VAPORIZING IS A HEALTHIER FORM OF INHALATION), WHEN THE MATERIAL STARTS TO TASTE BURNT OR LOOK DARK BROWN PLACE IT IN A JAR WITH A LID AND PUT IN A COOL DARK PLACE (CABINET). WHEN YOU HAVE SAVED ENOUGH OF THIS A.B.V MATERIAL IT IS COOKING TIME!

WHEN YOU VAPORIZE, YOU ARE HEATING UP THE PLANT TO WHERE ONLY THE CANNABINOIDS BURN. THERE IS NO COMBUSTION FROM THE PLANT MATERIAL MAKING THIS IS THE HEALTHIEST WAY TO INHALE. BECAUSE YOU HAVE BURNT OFF A LOT OF THE THC AND SOME OF THE OTHER CANNABINOIDS IT IS BEST TO USE HALF MORE OR DOUBLE THE AMOUNT YOU WOULD NORMALLY USE, THIS WILL ENSURE A POTENT AND EFFECTIVE PRODUCT.

OTHER TIPS AND SCIENTIFIC HEALTH BENEFITS OF CANNABIS

THC-A

THC-A (TETRAHYDROCANNABINOLIC ACID) IS FOUND IN THE RAW PLANT MATERIAL OF CANNABIS, THE CANNABIS BUD IS FULL OF THC-A, IT IS ONLY CONVERTED TO THC WITH HEAT.

THC-A IS VERY BENEFICIAL FOR INFLAMMATION. MOST CHRONIC PAIN CONDITIONS (EX. FIBROMYALGIA) ARE EFFECTED BY INFLAMMATION, SO IF YOU CAN TREAT THE INFLAMMATION THEN YOU CAN TREAT THE PAIN. WITH THC-A YOU ARE NOT ONLY TREATING THE INFLAMMATION AND PAIN YOU ARE ALSO PREVENTING ANY FLARE UPS, AND BECAUSE THC-A IS NON-PSYCHOACTIVE IT CAN BE CONSUMED IN LARGER DOSES.

THC-A IS ALSO VERY EFFECTIVE IN TREATING AND PREVENTING CERTAIN CANCERS, BECAUSE OF ITS ANTI-INFLAMMATORY PROPERTIES THC-A HELPS PREVENT CERTAIN CANCERS FROM SPREADING.

THE RESEARCH ON THC-A IS IN ITS INFANCY, HOWEVER IT IS PROVEN TO BE VERY EFFECTIVE FOR NEUROPATHY AND NAUSEA.

OTHER TIPS AND SCIENTIFIC
HEALTH BENEFITS OF CANNABIS

<u>CHLOROPHYLL</u>

CHLOROPHYLL IS A NATURAL BI-PRODUCT OF PLANTS. WHEN CONSUMED CHLOROPHYLL CAN HELP PROMOTE A HEALTHY IMMUNE SYSTEM, CLEANSE THE BODY, ENCOURAGE HEALING, CONTROL BODY ODORS, REDUCE NAUSEA AND MUCH MORE. THE CHLOROPHYLL FROM CANNABIS IS ALSO GREAT FOR INFLAMMATION AND PAIN PREVENTION.

WE RECOMMEND KEEPING THE CHLOROPYLL, HOWEVER, IF YOU WANT TO REMOVE CHLOROPHYLL FROM YOUR BUTTER YOU CAN DO SO BY ADDING ONE CUP OF WATER TO THE MELTED BUTTER IN THE DOUBLE BOILER AND FOLLOWING THE COOKING PROCEDURES FOR THE CANNA-BUTTER.

ONCE THE COOKING IS COMPLETE, STRAIN CANNA-BUTTER NORMALLY AND PLACE IN A HEAT SAFE STORAGE BOWL/JAR AND PUT IN THE FRIDGE FOR 4-6 HOURS (SOMETIMES TAKES LONGER) FOR COOLING.

OTHER TIPS AND SCIENTIFIC
HEALTH BENEFITS OF CANNABIS

CHLOROPHYLL *CONT'D*

🍁 WHEN THE MATERIAL IS COOLED, REMOVE FROM FRIDGE, THE TOP PART SHOULD BE GREEN AND SOLID AND THE BOTTOM SHOULD BE A DARK WATERY LIQUID.

🍁 GRAB A STRAINER AND SEPARATE THE GREEN BUTTER FROM THE LIQUID (BEING SURE NOT TO GET THE BUTTER DIRTY), CLEAN REMAINING "SLUDGE" OFF OF BUTTER WITH A PAPER TOWEL AND PLACE IN BOWL/JAR WITH A LID AND PUT IN FRIDGE.

OTHER TIPS AND SCIENTIFIC
HEALTH BENEFITS OF CANNABIS

EXTRACTS

WHEN COOKING WITH CANNABIS, YOU CAN USE PLANT MATERIAL OR CANNABIS EXTRACTS THAT WERE MADE FROM PLANT MATERIAL. THESE EXTRACTS ARE KNOWN AS HASH, WAX, SHATTER, DISTILLATE, KEIF, BATTER AND OTHER NAMES.

WHEN USING EXTRACTS YOU WONT NEED AS MUCH MATERIAL BECAUSE IT IS MORE CONCENTRATED, HOWEVER IT CAN BE PRICIER THEN BUYING THE PLANT MATERIAL. BECAUSE EXTRACTS ARE STRONGER, IT IS WISE TO APPROACH WITH CAUTION AND START OFF BY CONSUMING A SMALL AMOUNT AT FIRST OR GET YOUR MATERIAL TESTED. MOST EXTRACTS ABSORB INTO THE BUTTER AND OIL EASILY.

MOST EXTRACTS ARE 600-900 MG OF THC PER GRAM, AND THEY INFUSE INTO OILS AND BUTTERS VERY EASILY.

OTHER TIPS AND SCIENTIFIC
HEALTH BENEFITS OF CANNABIS

EXTRACTS *CONT'D*

🍁 BECAUSE OF THE STRENGTH, IT IS BEST TO KNOW HOW MANY MILLIGRAMS OR THC YOU ARE INFUSING INTO YOUR OIL. YOU CAN FIND THIS INFORMATION AT THE DISPENSARY YOU PURCHASED FROM AND THEN DO THE MATH OF HOW MANY MILLIGRAMS OF THC TO THE AMOUNT OF OIL YOU ARE INFUSING TO FIND OUT HOW MANY MG/ML OF OIL.

🍁 EXAMPLE:
1 GRAM OF OIL EQUALS 600-900 MG OF THC (WE WILL USE 900 MG AS THE EXAMPLE)

THERE ARE 8 OZ IN 1 CUP OF OIL OR BUTTER

THERE ARE 30 ML IN 1 OZ

900 MG / 8 OZ = 112.5 MG OF THC PER 1 OZ OF OIL

112.5 MG / 30 ML= 3.75 MG OF THC PER 1 ML OF OIL OR BUTTER.

1ml = 3.75 mg of THC

INFUSING OIL OR BUTTER WITH CANNABIS

MATERIALS NEEDED:

- 1/2LB OF BUTTER OR 8OZ OF OIL

- 3.5GM (1/8TH) DRIED AND CURED CANNABIS BUDS OR SHAKE (OR 7GM ABV), OR 1 GRAM OF EXTRACT

- CANNABIS GRINDER

- SAUCE PAN OR DOUBLE BOILER (FOR BUTTER)

- MEASURING CUP

- SPOON

- METAL STAINER

- THERMOMETER

- CHEESECLOTH

- BOWL OR JAR FOR STORAGE

- TONGS (OPTIONAL)

INFUSING OIL OR BUTTER WITH CANNABIS

THE PROCESS

*THERE MAY BE A STRONG SCENT OF CANNABIS WHILE INFUSING YOUR OIL, ESPECIALLY WHEN HEAT IS APPLIED TO CANNABIS.

- USE CANNABIS GRINDER TO GROUND UP CANNABIS, BE SURE NOT TO OVER GRIND, YOU DON'T WANT IT TO BE A FINE POWDER OR IT WILL BE HARDER TO STRAIN.

- PLACE SAUCE PAN WITH OIL OR DOUBLE BOILER WITH BUTTER ON LOW TO MEDIUM HEAT, IF USING A DOUBLE BOILER THE HEAT WILL BE HIGHER DUE TO THE WATER HAVING TO BOIL.

- ADD GROUNDED UP RAW CANNABIS (OR DECARBOXYLATED CANNABIS, OR EXTRACT) TO OIL OR BUTTER AND LET SIMMER AT A LOW TO MEDIUM HEAT FOR 20-30MIN. STIR EVERY 5 MINUTES AND CONSTANTLY

- CHECK TEMPERATURE WITH THERMOMETER, THIS IS THE CRUCIAL PART OF THE PROCESS BECAUSE YOU DON'T WANT YOUR PRODUCT TO BURN. KEEP AROUND 160-180°F, DO NOT EXCEED 225°F

INFUSING OIL OR BUTTER WITH CANNABIS

THE PROCESS *CONT'D*

✦ ONCE PRODUCT HAS COOKED FOR DESIRED AMOUNT OF TIME, REMOVE FROM HEAT AND LET COOL FOR 5 MINUTES. AFTER THE PRODUCT HAS COOLED FOR 5 MINUTES, USE METAL STRAINER AND CHEESECLOTH TO STRAIN THE FINISHED PRODUCT AND REMOVE ALL PLANT MATERIAL. (TIP: PUT CHEESECLOTH IN STRAINER AND POUR MATERIAL THROUGH INTO YOUR JAR OR BOWL.

✦ AFTER ALL MATERIAL HAS BEEN TRANSFERRED THROUGH CHEESECLOTH AND STRAINER, ROLL UP THE CHEESECLOTH IN THE STRAINER AND PUSH DOWN TO GET REMAINING OIL OR BUTTER OUT.) ***IF MATERIAL IS STILL HOT DURING STRAINING, YOU CAN USE TONGS TO SQUEEZE OUT EXCESS MATERIAL***

CONGRATULATIONS!!!
YOU JUST SUCCESSFULLY MADE CANNABIS INFUSED OIL OR BUTTER!!!

✦ NOW YOU CAN USE THIS MATERIAL TO MAKE EDIBLES, CAPSULES, TINTURES, OR EVEN TOPICALS. WE ARE FIRM BELIEVER IN TOPICALS LIKE NANA'S RUB, WHICH YOU CAN FIND AT SHOPCLEANHEMP.COM

✦ TOPICALS ARE THE ONLY WAY TO GET RELIEF IN AN EXACT AREA

✦ TO STORE, PUT LID ON JAR OR BOWL THAT CONTAINS THE FINISHED PRODUCT AND PLACE IN THE FRIDGE FOR YOUR CANNABIS COOKING NEEDS.

✦ CHECK YOUR BUTTER LABEL FOR EXPIRATION DATES, COCONUT OIL SHOULD LAST A WHILE.

✦ IF YOU ARE MAKING BUTTER, IT HELPS TO OBTAIN A BUTTER MOLD. BY USING THE MOLD YOU CAN POUR THE MELTED BUTTER IN AND IT WILL TAKE THE SHAPE OF A BUTTER STICK AGAIN, THIS MIGHT BE EASIER TO USE FOR COOKING.

✦ ENJOY ALL YOUR CANNA-INFUSED PRODUCTS AND ALWAYS CONSUME SAFELY!

THANK YOU FOR THE OPPORTUNITY TO HELP YOU.
LIVE WELL AND BE HAPPY!!!

CANNABIS SAVES LIVES!!!!

HOW TO MAKE THE EASIEST LOW HEAT CHOCOLATE EVER!!!

MATERIALS NEEDED:

- 4OZ CANNABIS COCONUT OIL

- ½ CUP COCOA POWDER (OR COCAO)

- ½ TSP OF SEA SALT

- 3 TBLS HONEY (OR MAPLE SYRUP)

- 1 ½ TBLS AGAVE NECTAR (OPTIONAL FOR SWEETER CHOCOLATE)

- ½ TSP VANILLA EXTRACT

- BOWL FOR MIXING

- WHISK

- ***CAN SUBSTITUTE 1 OZ OR 2 OZ OF COCONUT OIL FOR COCO BUTTER TO MAKE A HARDER CHOCOLATE BUT YOU WILL LOSE POTENCY***

HOW TO MAKE THE EASIEST CHOCOLATE EVER!!!

<u>THE PROCESS</u>

🍁 HEAT UP CANNA-OIL TO LOW TO MEDIUM HEAT (UNDER 180°F)

🍁 ADD IN COCOA POWDER, SEA SALT, VANILLA EXTRACT AND WHISK UNTIL ALL LUMPS ARE OUT AND CHOCOLATE IS SMOOTH

🍁 LET COOL FOR 10 MIN

🍁 ADD IN HONEY AND AGAVE NECTAR, WHISK UNTIL ALL LUMPS ARE OUT AND CHOCOLATE IS SMOOTH

🍁 POUR IN TO CHOCOLATE MOLDS AND PLACE IN FRIDGE, LET COOL FOR AT LEAST AN HOUR.

🍁 TAKE ONE OUT AND ENJOY!!!!!!

CONCLUSION

THANK YOU FOR THIS OPPORTUNITY TO HELP YOU LEARN MORE ABOUT CANANBIS AND IT'S BENEFITS.

AS WE CONTINUE TO LEARN MORE, WE WILL CONTINUE TO SHARE.

YOU CAN LEARN MORE ABOUT CANNABIS AND LISTEN/WATCH ANY PODCASTS BY GOING TO MMJDAVID.COM

CANNABIS IS A GATEWAY TO NATURAL MEDICINE AND SELF HEALING. NATURE PROVIDES ALL THAT WE NEED TO BE HEALTHY.

THIS IS A DAVID YRIGOYEN LLC PRODUCTION

DAVIDYRIGOYEN.COM

NOTES:

NOTES:

NOTES:

www.ingramcontent.com/pod-product-compliance
Lightning Source LLC
Chambersburg PA
CBHW052125030426
42335CB00025B/3129

9 798218 340964